TABLE OF CONTENTS

INTRODUCTION

A diagnosis of diabetes can be frightening. If you've only recently received a diagnosis, the task of managing your disease can seem especially daunting. But you don't need to be a prisoner of diabetes. You can actively participate in your own care, using the tools at your disposal, to feel better and enjoy improved health and well-being. You'll also lower your risk of diabetes complications. It takes dedication, but *You Can Reverse Diabetes* is here to help you tackle the task.

One tool at your disposal is information. Faced with a health problem, we sometimes want to bury our head in the sand. It's easier to avoid thinking about potential problems we may encounter, or lifestyle changes we may need to adopt. But the more you know, the better your chances at avoiding those potential problems.

Lifestyle changes, including changes to your diet and exercise routine, are some of the most powerful tools in your arsenal for reversing diabetes and diabetes-related problems. For some people, diabetes can be reversed completely with lifestyle changes alone. Others can slow or stop the progression of the disease, prevent or delay serious complications, and reduce or eliminate reliance on insulin and medications.

The Obesity-Diabetes Connection
Currently, more than one-third of American adults (34.9% or 78.6 million) are considered obese. Compared to adults who weigh a healthy amount, obese individuals are more than *seven times* as likely to develop diabetes. And the problem is not restricted to adults. An estimated 12.5 million kids in America today fall in the obese category. More than ever before, overweight children and teenagers are developing insulin resistance and type 2 diabetes.

No Coincidence
In a Gallup-Healthways survey conducted in 2012, six of the ten states with the highest obesity rates were also among the ten states with the highest rates of diabetes. Those states were (in alphabetical order): Alabama, Kentucky, Louisiana, Mississippi, Tennessee, and West Virginia.

Are You Overweight?
Stepping on the scale doesn't tell the whole story. Doctors use body mass index (BMI) to determine whether a person's weight is proportionate to their height. If your BMI falls between 25 and 29, you're overweight. If it's 30 or higher, you are considered obese.

Here's how to calculate your BMI:

1) Weigh yourself first thing in the morning, without clothes.
2) Confirm your height, in inches.
3) Multiply your weight in pounds by 700.
4) Divide the result in step 3 by your height in inches.
5) Divide the result in step 4 by your height in inches again.

The resulting number is your BMI.

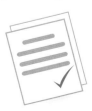

CHAPTER 1
Understanding the Problem

Knowledge is power, and the more you understand about diabetes, the better able you are to fight it. This first chapter provides an overview—what diabetes is, how it develops, and other important information—that will get you acquainted with what's going on in your body so that you can manage your condition as effectively as possible.

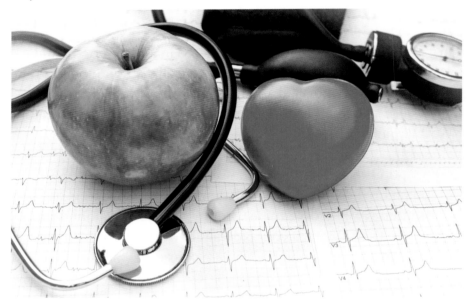

What Is Diabetes?

Diabetes is a problem with energy production. (In medical terms, it's a metabolic disorder.) High levels of sugar in the blood mark this chronic, progressive disease. Much of the food we eat is digested and converted into a type of sugar called glucose, which serves as the main fuel for the body's cells. To reach each cell, this sugary fuel travels through the bloodstream, which is why we refer to it as "blood sugar." Once there, it's normally greeted by insulin, a hormone made in the pancreas. Insulin acts as a sort of key that opens the cell's door to allow the vital sugar in.

In a person with diabetes, the body either produces little or no insulin, or the insulin can't do its job effectively because the cells don't respond to it the way they should. As a result, the cells go hungry while sugar continues to pile up in the bloodstream.

TYPES OF DIABETES

Type 1 Diabetes

If you have type 1 diabetes, the chances are pretty good that you have known it for a long time: Half of all people diagnosed with type 1 diabetes are younger than 20 years old. In fact, type 1 diabetes used to be called juvenile-onset diabetes, back before doctors realized that the condition could actually strike people of any age. Another name sometimes used is insulin-dependent diabetes, since virtually all folks with type 1 require injections of the crucial hormone insulin. In the United States, only about 5 percent of all people with diagnosed diabetes have type 1, making it far less common than type 2 diabetes.

Type 1 diabetes begins with a glitch in the immune system, the body's defense against bacteria, viruses, and other unwanted invaders that try to make you sick. The immune system is a complex network of vessels, fluids, white blood cells, and special proteins called antibodies that patrol your innards, looking for things that don't belong. When your immune system detects a germ or anything else that it doesn't recognize as belonging to the body, it fires off white blood cells and antibodies to engulf and destroy the intruder.

Unfortunately, in some people the immune system is guilty of friendly fire. It mistakes perfectly innocent and otherwise healthy body tissue for an enemy invader, attacking it with an onslaught of voracious immune cells. Depending on what part of the body your immune system attacks, the result can be one of many

Type I diabetes

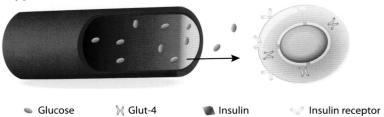

| Glucose | Glut-4 | Insulin | Insulin receptor |

autoimmune diseases, which include rheumatoid arthritis, lupus, thyroiditis, and type 1 diabetes.

In someone with type 1 diabetes, the immune system mistakenly destroys the cells in the pancreas that make insulin, known as beta cells. The body treats these cells as invaders and destroys them. As beta cells die off, insulin production slows down or even stops. Since the pancreas is the only part of the body that can produce insulin, an autoimmune attack on the organ leaves the body without this essential hormone.

With no insulin available, most of the body's cells are unable to get the sugar they need to survive, even though there is a great deal of it floating around in the bloodstream. To survive, people with type 1 diabetes require insulin injections to control blood sugar levels.

The exact causes of type 1 diabetes are not yet known. If you have type 1 diabetes, there's a good chance one of your parents passed along to you an abnormal gene or cluster of genes that puts you at greater-than-average risk for developing the condition. But being born with these genes doesn't guarantee that you will develop type 1 diabetes. These inherited genes only make you *susceptible* to developing diabetes. Something else has to trigger changes in your body to create your blood sugar problem. But what?

Scientists aren't sure, but they have a short list of suspects. According to one theory, a virus or some environmental toxin worms its way into the body and confuses the immune system because it resembles proteins found on beta cells. The immune system tends to shoot first and ask questions later, so it destroys anything that looks like it could be a threat—including insulin-producing beta cells in the pancreas. Type 1 diabetes occurs more often in people who have had a viral illness, as this can trigger the onset of type 1 diabetes in a susceptible individual.

Type II diabetes

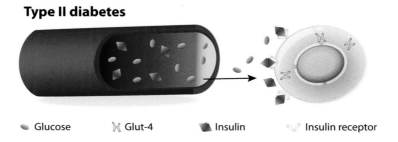

● Glucose   ✕ Glut-4   ◤ Insulin   ◡ Insulin receptor

Type 2 Diabetes

Approximately 90–95 percent of people with diagnosed diabetes in the United States have type 2. Like type 1 diabetes, this condition used to go by other names, including non-insulin-dependent diabetes and adult-onset diabetes. Now it's clear that both terms are misnomers. A person with type 2 diabetes may indeed be insulin dependent, and type 2 isn't limited to adults, either.

Unlike type 1, type 2 diabetes is not an autoimmune disease, in which the body attacks its own cells. Type 2 diabetes usually starts as "insulin resistance," a disorder in which the body's cells become less and less able to respond to insulin, causing the sugar level in the blood to rise. In an effort to push sugar into the body's still-hungry cells, the pancreas churns out more and more insulin, increasing the level of insulin in the blood even while the blood sugar level remains high. Over time, the exhausted pancreas begins to lose its ability to produce sufficient insulin.

Insulin resistance causes no symptoms. It's not as though you can feel or hear glucose molecules crashing into your resistant, tightly closed cells. However, insulin resistance often sets the stage for type 2 diabetes. Bottom line: If you have type 2 diabetes, you almost certainly have insulin resistance.

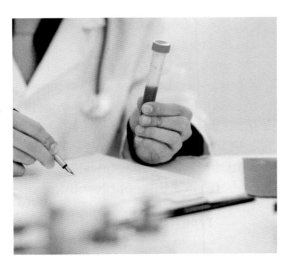

It usually takes insulin resistance months or years to progress to type 2 diabetes, when beta cells become progressively incapable of meeting the demand for insulin. At that point, insulin levels in the blood rise, too, as the beta cells keep cranking out the hormone in an attempt to coax open stubborn cells.

Type 2 diabetes is more common in people who are significantly overweight or obese and those who engage in little or no physical activity. Family history also plays a major role. Having close relatives with type 2 diabetes greatly increases your risk of the disease. Certain ethnic groups, including Native Americans, African Americans, Hispanic Americans, Asian Americans, and Pacific Islanders are also at high risk. The aging process plays a role, too. The older we get, the more insulin resistant we tend to become, so the risk of developing type 2 diabetes increases with age.

Type 2 diabetes is treated with lifestyle changes, oral medications, and insulin. Some people with type 2 can control their blood glucose with healthy eating and being active. But oral medications or insulin may also be needed. Type 2 diabetes is a progressive disease, so even if you don't need medications at first, you may need them later on.

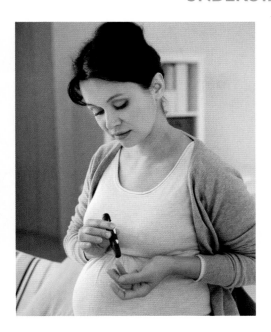

Gestational Diabetes

Gestational diabetes may affect anywhere from 2–18 percent of pregnancies. The condition usually doesn't arise until after 20 weeks of pregnancy. And while any pregnant woman can develop gestational diabetes, it's more common among those who:

• Are older than 25

• Have a parent or sibling with diabetes

• Are African American, American Indian, Asian American, Hispanic American, or Pacific Islander

• Are overweight

• Developed gestational diabetes during a previous pregnancy or have given birth to an infant who weighed more than nine pounds

• Have ever been told by a doctor that they have prediabetes, impaired glucose tolerance, or impaired fasting glucose

So what's the harm in having high blood sugar for a few months? For starters, women with gestational diabetes often develop high blood pressure (referred to as pre-eclampsia), which brings its own risks for both mother and baby. What's more, they frequently give birth to very large babies who weigh more than nine pounds. Not only do fat babies often require a caesarean-section delivery, they're also more likely to be fat children and to develop diabetes by their teen years or young adulthood (because of their genetic inheritance, not the intrauterine environment).

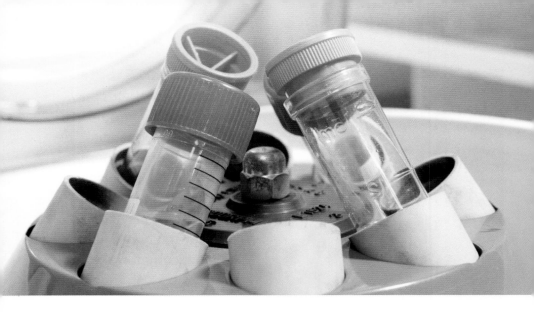

The news about gestational diabetes isn't all bad. After all, there's a reliable cure for the problem: having your baby, after which most women's blood sugar levels return to normal. However, the condition lingers in a small number of women, who are then diagnosed with either type 1 or type 2 diabetes. Regardless, if you have gestational diabetes once, the odds are two out of three that you'll develop it again with a subsequent pregnancy. More concerning, women who have gestational diabetes stand a 20–50 percent risk of developing type 2 diabetes within a decade.

Prediabetes
Prediabetes is the most common form of diabetes. It has been estimated that about 86 million Americans aged 20 years and older have prediabetes. People with prediabetes have blood glucose (sugar) levels that are higher than normal—but not high enough to be diagnosed as diabetes. Prediabetes can lead to heart disease, stroke, and type 2 diabetes. Most people who have prediabetes develop full-blown type 2 diabetes within 10 years. Prediabetes can often be reversed with diet and exercise.

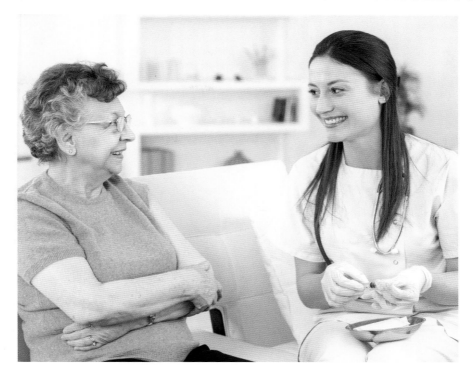

Double Diabetes

Although it's not a term you will find in most medical textbooks, many doctors today say they are treating a growing number of type 1 diabetes patients who have also developed insulin resistance, the classic symptom of type 2 diabetes. Some doctors are treating these hybrid patients with drugs that make their bodies more sensitive to insulin. The term "double diabetes" may also be used to describe a person with type 2 diabetes who develops antibodies that destroy the pancreatic beta cells (the ones that produce insulin); in most cases, these patients will require insulin injections. Just to make matters more confusing, double diabetes is sometimes called type 3 diabetes.

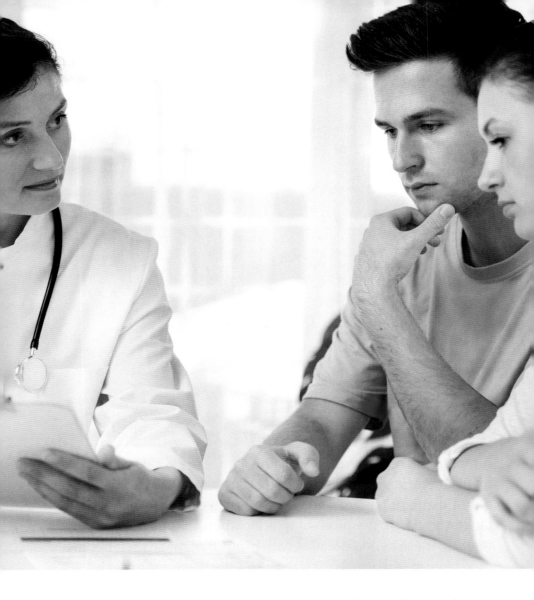

Latent Autoimmune Diabetes of Adulthood (LADA)

LADA is also known as slow-onset type 1 diabetes. About 5–10 percent of people with diabetes are adults who develop the type 1 variety of the condition, which is typically first diagnosed in children and teens. Doctors often mistake the condition for plain old type 2 diabetes, basing their diagnosis solely on a patient's age and high blood sugar. But people with LADA don't have insulin resistance and aren't necessarily overweight. Those are important distinctions, since they influence which treatments work for LADA.

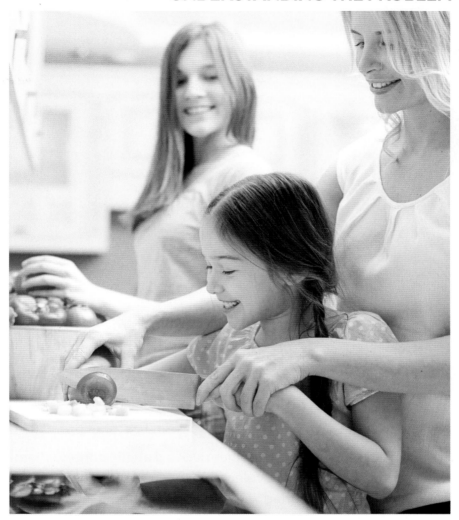

Maturity-Onset Diabetes of the Young (MODY)

MODY is something like the flipside of LADA. It usually turns up in teens and young adults, although it may be found in children as well as older adults. Because patients tend to be youngish and slender, doctors often misdiagnose the condition as type 1 diabetes. However, MODY is a genetic disorder that interferes with insulin production. And unlike people with type 2 diabetes, those with MODY don't have insulin resistance. Again, getting the right diagnosis is critical in order to choose the proper treatment approach for MODY.

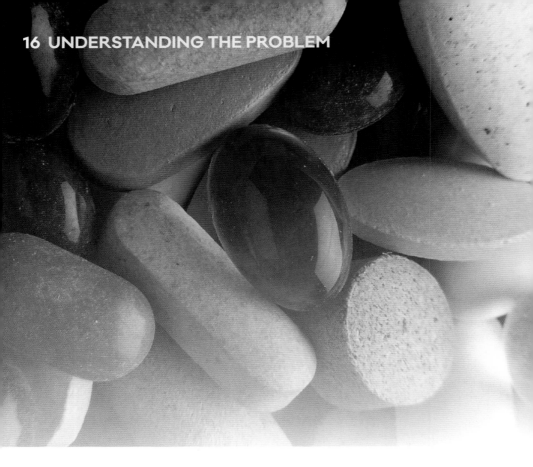

Secondary Diabetes

Certain diseases and drug therapies pack a diabetic double wham-my by making people more vulnerable to blood sugar problems, either by directly interfering with insulin or by producing physical changes that increase insulin resistance (such as weight gain) and can lead to diabetes. When another identifiable medical prob-lem or medication precipitates the development of diabetes, it is called secondary diabetes. A brief list of conditions that may cause secondary diabetes includes depression, HIV, pancreatitis, certain hormonal disorders (such as Cushing's syndrome and hyper-thyroidism), and some genetic disorders (such as cystic fibrosis). Drugs linked to secondary diabetes include diuretics and other drugs used to treat high blood pressure, steroid hormones, certain asthma medications, antidepressants, anticonvulsants, and some forms of cancer chemotherapy, among others.

CHAPTER 2
Fighting Diabetes with Food

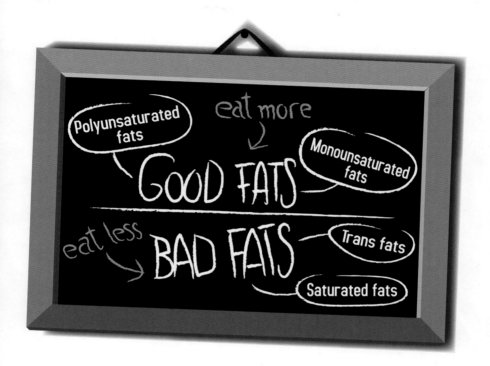

A sound eating plan is one of the most powerful tools you have to fight diabetes and diabetes-related complications. Your diet should be high in fiber, rich in omega-3 fatty acids, and include colorful fresh fruits and vegetables with phytonutrients (natural substances found in plants that help protect the plant from disease). In humans, phytonutrients such as carotenoids, flavonoids, and polyphenols are associated with a lower incidence of nearly all health problems, including obesity and age-related disease.

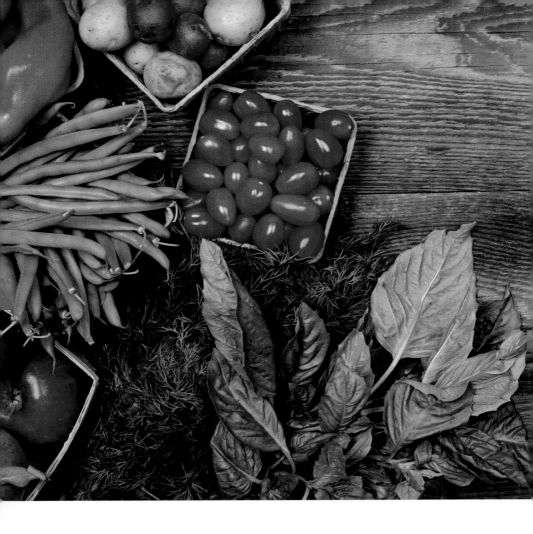

Get Colorful

One way to add variety to your diet is to add more foods with an array of different colors. Nutritionists believe that the same chemicals that give certain kinds of fruits and vegetables a brilliant hue may also promote health and fight disease. Tomatoes and watermelon, for example, get their red color from an antioxidant called lycopene, which may prevent some cancers. You may want to see green on your plate, in particular. Some researchers believe that the antioxidants lutein and zeaxanthin, which are found in spinach, collards, kale, and broccoli, may strengthen the retina, the ring of nerve cells in the eyes that are vulnerable to blinding damage from high blood sugar.

Substituting Good Fats for Bad Fats

1. Cook with olive oil. If you need flavorless oil, try canola or grapeseed oil. If the recipe requires the rich taste of butter, you can usually replace half of it with oil without compromising flavor.

2. Change your dressing. Store-bought salad dressings can be loaded with sugar or preservatives. Make a simple vinaigrette with olive oil, or just pass a good quality vinegar and olive oil at the table.

3. Avoid processed meat. It can hide bad fat and sometimes bad carbs, too.

4. Choose low-fat dairy. Drink low-fat milk. Watch out for cheese. It can contribute a lot of fat to food, most of it saturated. Try using small amounts of full-flavored cheeses like Parmesan.

5. Cook at home. Deep-fried chicken, potatoes, and fish from restaurants are very likely to contain high levels of trans fats. Home-cooked meals are almost always healthier.

6. Go fish. Fatty fish, such as salmon, tuna, and sardines, contain beneficial omega-3 fatty acids. These fats appear to improve cholesterol.

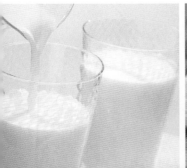
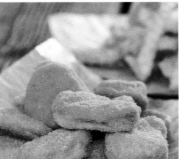
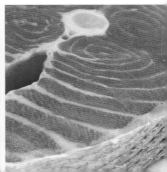

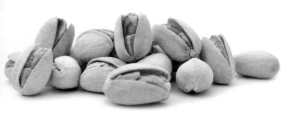

FOODS IN THE SPOTLIGHT

On these pages, we'll focus the spotlight on some specific foods that you can try to help prevent, manage, treat, and reverse diabetes.

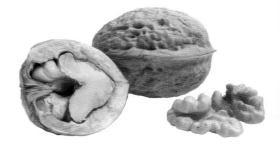

Nuts and Seeds

An ounce of nuts can go a long way in providing key healthy fats along with hunger management. Other benefits are a dose of magnesium and fiber.

Walnuts are especially helpful for people with type 2 diabetes, when eaten in moderation. They've been shown to reduce common dangerous characteristics of the disease, including insulin resistance, excess body weight, and increased risk of heart disease. Walnuts provide a hefty amount of alpha-linolenic acid, the plant-based source of omega-3 fats that helps prevent blood clotting, reduce inflammation, and lower triglyceride levels in the blood. Walnuts also supply protein and soluble fiber, a combination of nutrients that helps to satisfy hunger, lower cholesterol, and smooth out blood sugar fluctuations.

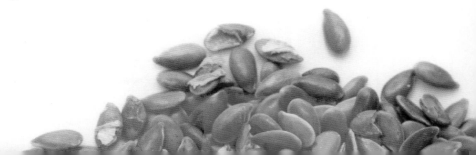

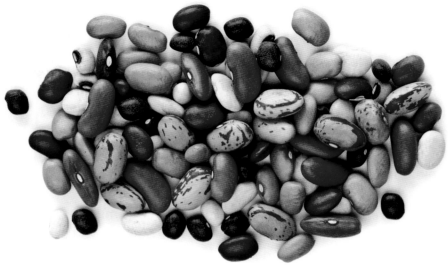

Beans

Lowly legumes are among the healthiest foods on the planet. They're packed with filling fiber, protein, B vitamins, and other nutrients. On average, beans contain 5 to 7 grams of fiber per ½ cup. Eating a mere 3 cups a week can help reduce the risk of heart disease and certain cancers. The soluble fiber in beans slows digestion and blunts the rise of blood sugar after meals. Most notably, their protein content makes them a perfect, nearly fat-free meat alternative. Beans come in a kaleidoscope of colors and shapes and are an important part of most every cuisine. From Asia's soybeans to Italy's cannellini beans to Mexico's pintos, beans offer many delectable options.

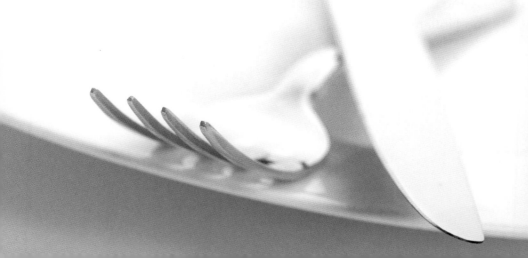

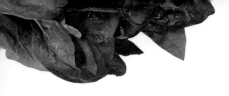

Leafy Greens

Leafy greens spinach, collards, and kale are low in calories and carbohydrate and rich in antioxidants. Cooked greens, such as collard greens, dandelion greens, mustard greens, turnip greens, and Swiss chard are a perfect side dish for many meals. They are hearty, flavorful, and packed with nutrients, especially vitamin A, vitamin C, iron, and calcium.

Spinach is reasonably high in fiber, offering twice as much as most other cooking or salad greens. This calorie-free bulk fills you up and keeps you feeling full longer, a great advantage if you're pursuing weight loss to improve your condition. Spinach also contains the phytonutrient lipoic acid, which assists energy production and may help regulate blood sugar. Where spinach really shines is as a source of essential antioxidant vitamins A, C, and E, and minerals manganese, selenium, and zinc.

Swiss chard provides an array of phytonutrients that may play a role in blocking the breakdown of carbohydrates into sugars, helping to prevent blood sugar from spiking following meals. The fiber and protein in Swiss chard also help to keep blood sugar on a more even keel by regulating the speed of digestion. And Swiss chard is loaded with antioxidant nutrients, including vitamins A and C, which help protect the body's cells from stress and inflammation.

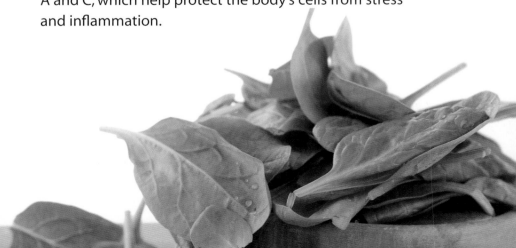

Citrus Fruits

Citrus fruits such as oranges, lemons, and limes provide fiber and are packed with vitamin C, which is essential for controlling infections. That is especially important for people with diabetes, who are at increased risk for a variety of infections. As an antioxidant, vitamin C also helps fight inflammation, which is suspected of playing a role not only in the development of diabetes, but in its progression and complications.

Oranges provide insoluble fiber to help with blood sugar control and also pack nutrients that battle diabetes complications. One orange provides 130 percent of the daily requirement for vitamin C, which helps control infections, maintain healthy teeth and gums, and protect small blood vessels. As an antioxidant, vitamin C works with the folate and potassium found in oranges to slow the development of coronary heart disease. Additionally, vitamin C and the orange-related phytochemical beta-carotene support eye health and lower the risk of sight-stealing cataracts.

Lemons are loaded with vitamin C. Lemons' zest, or outer skin, is rich in another antioxidant, rutin, which may help strengthen blood vessel walls and protect them from damage.

Limes provide a ton of flavor for very few calories and carbohydrates. Additionally, the powerful phytochemicals found in limes may help protect cells from damage that can lead to heart disease.

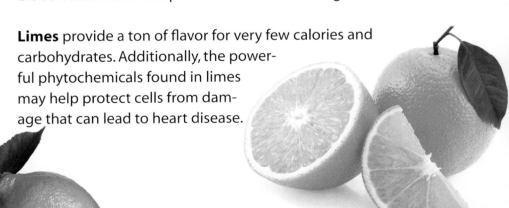

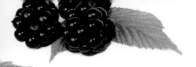

Berries

All berries are packed with antioxidants, vitamins, and fiber.

Blueberries are antioxidant superstars, ranking second among top antioxidant-rich foods. These flavorful berries are great for your eyes, memory, and heart. Blueberries are a good source of fiber and also provide vitamin C and iron. Recent research suggests that eating blueberries as part of a healthy diet may help reduce several key risk factors for cardiovascular disease and diabetes, such as accumulation of belly fat, high blood cholesterol, and high blood sugar. Antioxidants in blueberries may also protect your eyes and brain cells and help reverse age-related memory loss.

Strawberries are rich in a variety of phytonutrients that protect the heart and assist in blood sugar control. Recent research found that the polyphenols in strawberries may have the ability to blunt a rise in blood sugar levels after consuming table sugar. Eating strawberries several times a week also appears to be associated with a lower risk of type 2 diabetes. Strawberries are an exceptional source of vitamin C; they contain more than oranges and grapefruit.

Blackberries are an excellent source of vitamin C. Even more notable is their fiber; a handful of them has more fiber than a serving of some whole grain cereals. They are packed with soluble fiber, which slows absorption of sugar and helps steady blood sugar levels. Their nearly black appearance comes from high levels of anthocyanins and ellagic acid, two phytonutrients with numerous health benefits, such as helping to prevent heart disease and cancer and combating aging.

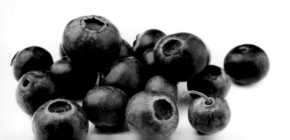

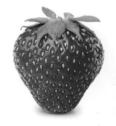

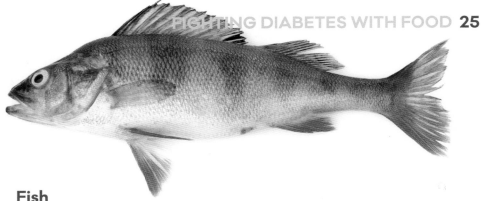

Fish

Fish is a smart catch for any diet. Eating at least two servings of fish each week offers multiple health benefits of special value to people with diabetes, such as improving the body's handling of blood sugar and warding off diseases of the heart, kidneys, and eyes—organs particularly vulnerable to damage from high blood sugar. Fish contain omega-3 fats and reduce inflammation, which can help counteract some of the negative effects of elevated blood glucose. Fish rich in essential omega-3 fatty acids include salmon, mackerel, rainbow trout, Albacore tuna, whitefish, halibut, sardines, anchovies, bass, and ocean perch. Omega-3s may also stimulate secretion of leptin, a hormone that helps regulate food intake, body weight, and metabolism.

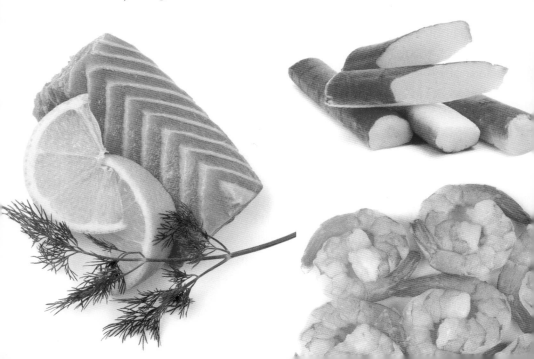

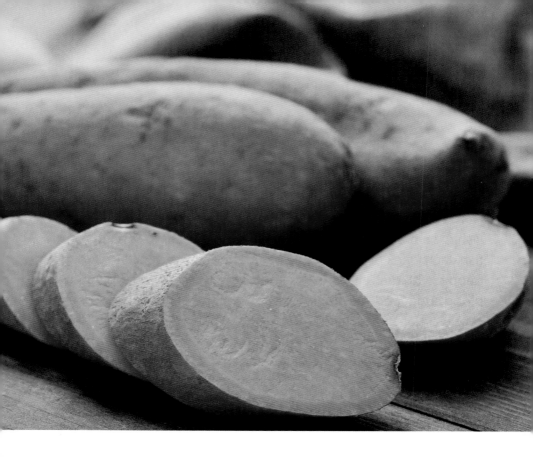

Sweet Potatoes

Their name may contain the word "sweet," but these root vegetables aren't high in sugar. They're extremely nutrient-rich and are often ranked as one of the healthiest foods. The carotenoids in sweet potatoes appear to help stabilize blood sugar levels due to their ability to lower insulin resistance by making cells more responsive to the hormone. These effects not only aid in disease management, but also make it easier to drop the excess pounds, which tend to aggravate the disease. Sweet potatoes also offer fiber to keep you full for hours. Furthermore, the hefty nutrient profile can help protect your heart and the rest of your body from damage and complications related to diabetes. For example, they supply infection-fighting vitamin C and blood pressure-lowering potassium.

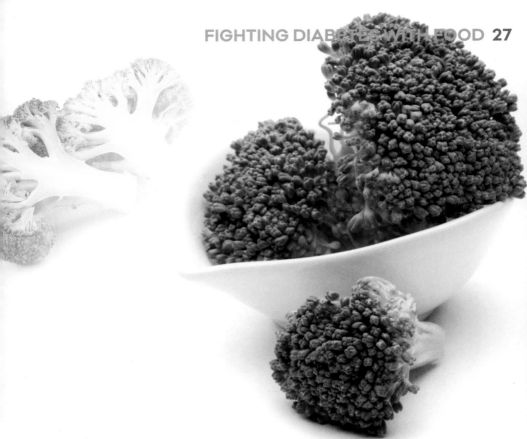

Broccoli

You are truly getting a powerhouse of nutrients when you incorporate this cruciferous vegetable into your diet. Broccoli's noteworthy nutrients include vitamin C, vitamin A (mostly as the antioxidant beta-carotene), folate, calcium, and fiber. It's a great nutritional bargain for a diabetes meal plan because in addition to being low in fat and calories, it's one of the vegetables lowest in sugars and carbohydrates. Broccoli is rich in an array of phytonutrients that serve as powerful cancer fighters, helping to inhibit tumor growth and boost the action of protective enzymes.

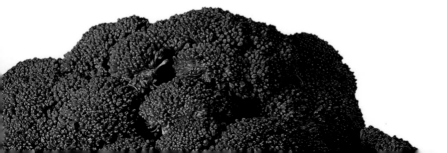

CHAPTER 3
Defeating Diabetes with Exercise

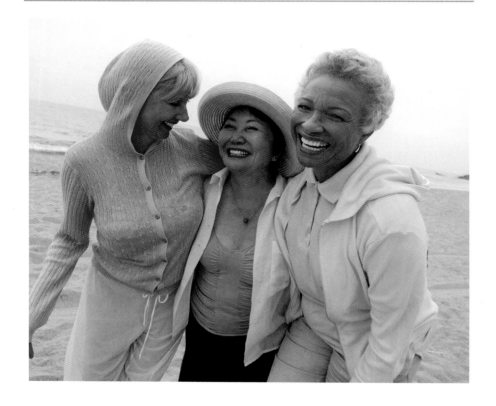

You may not think of a brisk walk, a game of tennis, or an hour spent cleaning your house as medicine for treating diabetes, but it is. Regular exercise is a potent tool for lowering blood sugar because it improves the way insulin works. Physical activity is also a proven way to combat conditions that often affect people with diabetes: heart disease, high blood pressure, infection, elevated cholesterol, depression, and increased stress. It burns extra calories—an important added benefit for those who need to lose weight. Physical activity also produces chemical messengers called endorphins that help relieve anxiety and pain. In short, exercise is one of the most effective tools you can use to combat diabetes.

Exercise and Type 1

For people with type 1 diabetes, timing is everything when it comes to exercise. Physical activity lowers blood sugar—the longer and more vigorous the workout, the lower blood sugar can drop—so taking steps to make sure the time is right to exercise will help you avoid hypoglycemia. As long as your blood sugar is under control and complications don't limit your mobility or tolerance for exercise, there's no need to sit on the bench. Just follow some simple rules.

1. Avoid vigorous activity if your fasting glucose is above 250 mg/dl and you test positive for ketones.

2. Exercise with caution if your fasting glucose is above 300 mg/dl in the absence of ketosis.

3. Consume carbs before exercising if your glucose level is below 100 mg/dl.

4. Monitor blood sugar before, during, and after exercise. Comparing the results will provide important information about how exercise affects your insulin needs. Based on how your blood sugar changes after a workout, your doctor or diabetes educator will recommend necessary changes to your insulin dose and provide advice about whether you need to consume carbs before exercising. Since you will probably respond differently to a 30-minute swim than a 60-minute walk, be sure to do before-and-after testing for all the different activities you participate in.

5. Keep glucose tablets or another carb source handy in case you become hypoglycemic.

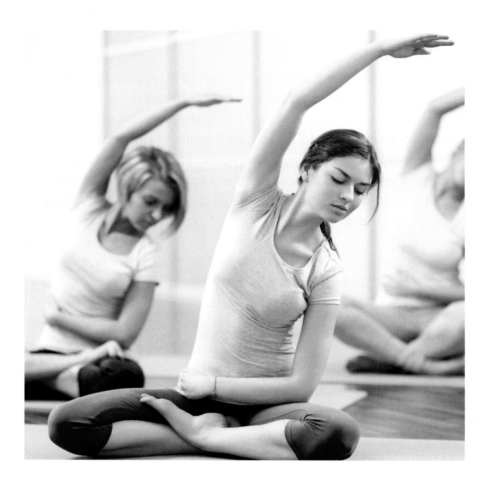

Exercise and Type 2

Exercise is a powerful tool for lowering blood sugar, because it improves insulin sensitivity. As discussed earlier, insulin resistance is an underlying cause of type 2 diabetes. For people with type 2 diabetes, it is possible to improve insulin sensitivity permanently by losing weight and keeping it off, and getting active can help with that. By incorporating regular exercise into their lives, many people with type 2 can increase their insulin sensitivity enough that they no longer need insulin injections or diabetes pills. And for folks who have been diagnosed with prediabetes, it is actually possible to prevent the full-blown disease through physical activity. The more calories the at-risk person burns per week by exercising, the lower their chances of progressing to type 2 diabetes!

Incorporating Activity

Take steps to incorporate more movement in your daily life. Especially if you've been a couch potato of late, those first steps toward becoming more active don't even have to look like exercise in the traditional sense. Being physically active every day means taking every opportunity you can to move more. Walking is a great way to start, and pedometers and fitness trackers can add motivation. Research has shown that people who wear pedometers and check them periodically throughout the day are motivated to walk and move more. Here are some simple ways to incorporate movement into your daily life:

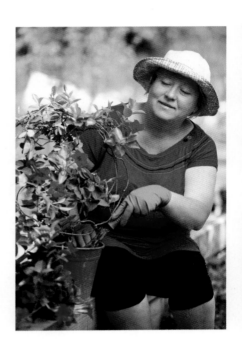

• Get in the habit of walking while you talk on the phone.

• When you go shopping, park farther away from the store's entrance.

• Take the stairs instead of elevators and escalators, particularly when going only one or two levels.

• At work, if you need to talk to a colleague on the other side of the building, walk instead of calling or e-mailing.

• If you have a dog, volunteer to be the person who walks it.

• Don't just sit in front of the TV. Hide the TV remote and get up to change channels. Buy a treadmill, stair-stepper, or small elliptical machine, and use it while you watch TV.

• Do your own yard work.

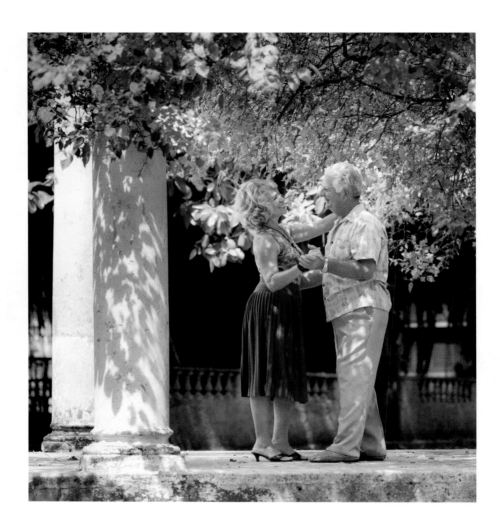

Developing an Exercise Routine

Once you begin adding more movement into your daily routine, the next step—establishing an exercise routine—will come much easier. Since you are looking to incorporate exercise into your daily routine, the activity you choose should also be something that you enjoy, that you have easy access to, and that is safe and reasonable for you to perform given your current health, abilities, and schedule. Your selection will also need a thumbs-up from your doctor, especially if you haven't been active recently.

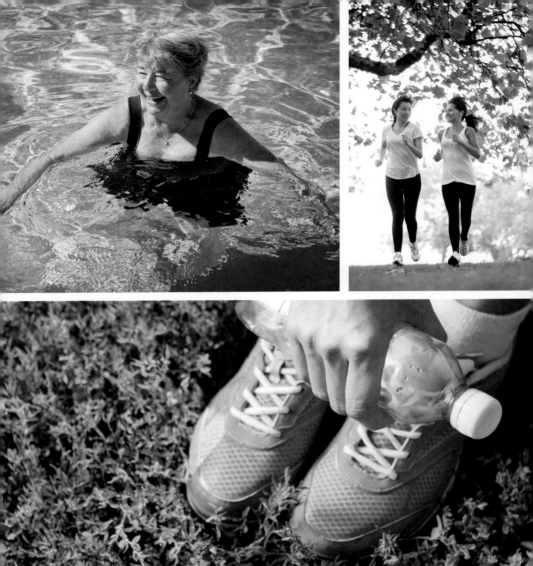

Besides deciding on a type of exercise, you also need to consider when you will exercise, how often, for how long, and how intensely. If you have an exercise physiologist on your diabetes care team, you can work together to devise an effective, challenging, and safe exercise program that evolves as your fitness increases.

Guidelines for Activity

• **See your physician** for a complete medical exam before adopting a new workout regimen.

• Choose activities that **fit your physical condition, lifestyle, and tastes.** Many people who have not been physically active for a while find that easy, low-impact activities such as walking and swimming are perfect.

• Make sure that whatever activities you choose are **enjoyable for you.** That increases the likelihood that you'll stick with it.

• **Vary your activities** so you don't get bored and fall prey to excuses. Choose some activities that can be done indoors in case of bad weather. Select some activities that can fit into a busy schedule.

• **Don't skimp** on exercise gear and equipment. Good-quality equipment pays for itself in the form of better protection against injuries. That's especially true for footwear. And always wear socks to keep your feet dry.

• **Warm up and cool down.** Begin each exercise session with a five- to ten-minute period of low-intensity activity and gentle stretching. This prepares your heart for increased activity. It also gives your muscles and joints a little time to get warm and loose. End your workouts with ten minutes of cool-down and more gentle stretching.

• Increase the amount of physical activity you do and its intensity slowly and **build up gradually**.

• Stay hydrated. **Drink plenty of water** before, during, and after exercise. Dehydration can spoil a good workout.

• **Identify yourself**. Just to be safe, always wear a bracelet, necklace, or shoe tag identifying yourself as a person with diabetes when you work out.

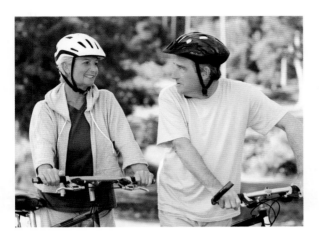

Low-Impact vs. High-Impact Activities

Another factor you'll want to consider is whether an activity is low-impact or high-impact. Low-impact activities are ones that don't involve a lot of jumping, pounding, or hitting anything with a lot of force, which can damage muscles, bones, and joints. If you haven't exercised regularly in some time, starting with low-impact activities can be a good idea. Swimming, cycling, hiking, and using an elliptical trainer all qualify as low-impact.

Those who have problems in their lower extremities would want to incorporate non-weight-bearing exercises such as stationary cycling, water exercise, and upper-body weight lifting. This includes anyone with very poor circulation or loss of nerve sensation in the legs or feet, as well as those with injuries, infections, or problems with balance.

If your fitness level allows, however, you can definitely enjoy higher-impact activities (such as running, jumping rope, boxing, or martial arts). If you have concerns, talk to your diabetes care team.

LOW-IMPACT ACTIVITIES

- Swimming
- Cycling
- "Power walking"
- Hiking
- Rowing
- Stair climbing
- Using an elliptical trainer
- Dancing
- Water aerobics

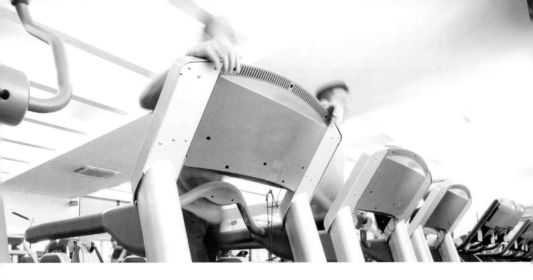

Intensity

How intensely should you exercise? Since your body is like no one else's, you'll need your own personal guide to tell you where to begin and how much physical effort you need to put in. Your best bet? Follow your heart. Your heart rate can tell you when you're working hard enough to increase your aerobic fitness.

Exercise physiologists have figured out a heart rate that is safe for most people during exercise. They call this your target heart-rate range. So what is your target heart rate? The following table can act as a guide.

YOUR AGE	TEN-SECOND TARGET HEART-RATE RANGE DURING EXERCISE
20–29	20–26
30–39	19–25
40–49	18–23
50–59	17–22
60–69	16–21
70–79	15–19
80+	14–18

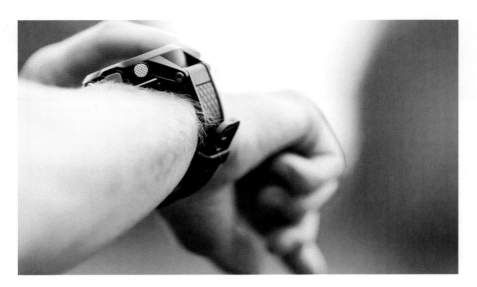

How to Measure Your Pulse

To check your heart rate, you need a watch that measures seconds, not just minutes. You can take your pulse either at the radial artery in your wrist (on the inner side of your wrist, below the heel of your hand) or the carotid artery in your neck. Use the index and middle fingers of one hand to feel the pulse. If you use the artery in your neck, however, place your fingers gently; putting too much pressure on this artery can actually slow down your pulse and give you a false reading. When you've found your pulse, count the number of beats for ten seconds.

Check your pulse as you continue the activity, if possible; otherwise, stop only long enough to count the heartbeats. Counting your pulse for ten seconds will let you know if you are above, below, or within your target heart-rate range.

If your heart rate during exercise is above the range listed in the table on page 36, slow down. If it is below, speed up a bit. Keep in mind that even if you maintain the same intensity, your heart rate may increase during the course of a workout as you begin to fatigue, so check your pulse every five or ten minutes throughout a longer workout to ensure you're still in your target range.

WORDS OF CAUTION

Although all people with diabetes should strive to be physically active, some forms of exercise require extra precautions (or may be too risky, period) for people who have any of the following complications.

Autonomic Neuropathy

Patients who have this form of nerve damage may not be able to detect symptoms such as sweating and rapid heart rate that signal the onset of exercise-induced hypoglycemia. They also have a high risk for orthostatic hypotension (a drop in blood pressure that can cause dizziness or fainting) during exercise performed while upright, so cycling or swimming may be better choices than walking or running. Beware of exercising in very hot or cold climates, and drink plenty of water.

Retinopathy

Some types of physical activity increase the risk of a hemorrhage in the eye or a detached retina. Avoid activities that involve a lot of jarring or straining, such as jogging or weight lifting.

Peripheral Neuropathy

If you can't feel your feet, how will you know if you're pounding the pavement too hard? People with serious loss of sensation in the lower limbs should not overdo weight-bearing exercise. Repetitive, intense pressure on the feet can cause ulcers. You may also fail to realize that you have broken a foot bone. If you have nerve damage that limits feeling in your feet, low-impact exercise, such as swimming, cycling, or rowing, may be the best choice.

CHAPTER 4
Aerobic Exercises

MARCH IN PLACE

Marching in place is a low-intensity, moderate-impact exercise. Like other aerobic activities, it increases the heart rate to strengthen the heart and lungs while also increasing circulation throughout the body. If neuropathy of the feet is present, do seated.

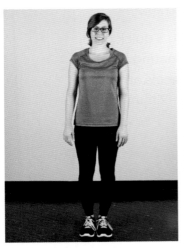

STEP 1
Stand (or sit) tall with abdominals pulled in.

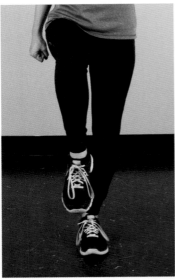
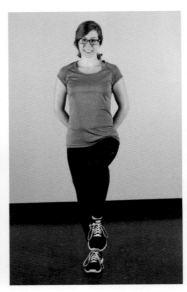

STEP 2
March in place for 1–2 minutes.

STEP 3
For added intensity, swing arms.

HEEL TAPS

Heel taps are a low-intensity, low-impact exercise. Along with providing cardiovascular benefits, heel taps also aid in stretching the back of legs and ankles.

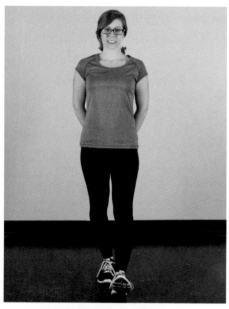

STEP 1
Stand (or sit) tall with abdominals pulled in.

Using a quick pace, alternating legs, tap heels on floor for 1–2 minutes.

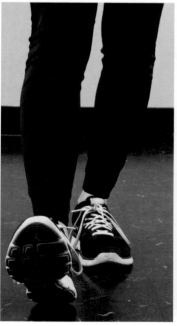

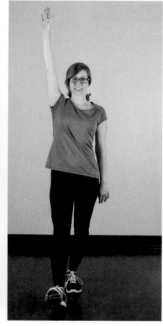

STEP 2
As you do this exercise, keep toe pointed to ceiling.

STEP 3
For added intensity, add an arm reach to ceiling.

RUN IN PLACE

Running in place is a moderate-intensity, moderate-impact aerobic exercise. Avoid this exercise if neuropathy of the feet is present.

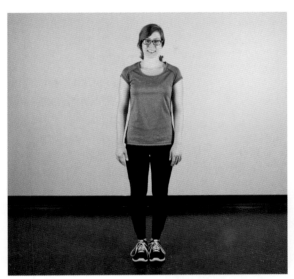

STEP 1
Stand tall with abdominals pulled in.

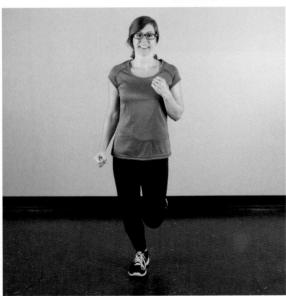

STEP 2
Run in place for 1–2 minutes.

STEP 3
For added intensity, swing arms.

HIGH KNEES

High knees are a moderate-intensity, moderate-impact exercise. Along with providing cardiovascular benefits, high knees also aids in strengthening the hip and core muscles. If neuropathy of the feet is present, do seated.

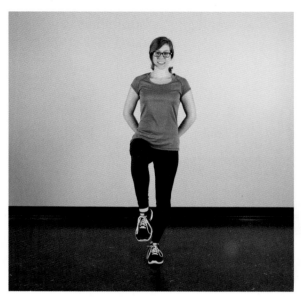

STEP 1
Stand (or sit) tall with abdominals pulled in.

Alternating legs, pull knees to hip level.

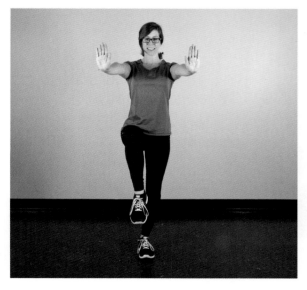

STEP 2
As you do this exercise, keep spine straight. Lift knees for 1–2 minutes.

STEP 3
For added intensity, add a forward press with arms.

SIDE STEPS

Side steps are a low-intensity, moderate-impact exercise. Along with providing cardiovascular benefits, side steps strengthen the outer and inner thighs. If neuropathy of the feet is present, do seated.

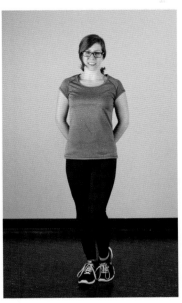

STEP 1

Stand (or sit) tall with abdominals pulled in.

Step both feet to the left and then step both feet to the right.

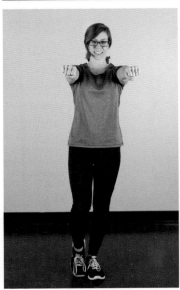

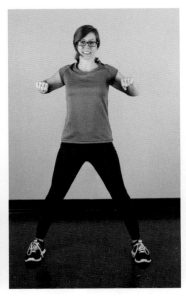

STEP 2

Step side to side for 1–2 minutes.

For added intensity, add a pulling movement with arms.

FORWARD AND BACK STEP

Stepping forward and back is a low-intensity, moderate-impact exercise. Along with providing cardiovascular benefits, stepping forward and back aids in training the walking and balance muscles of the upper leg. If neuropathy of the feet is present, do seated.

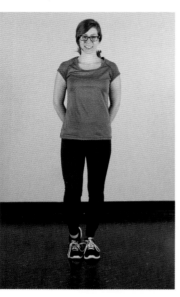

STEP 1
Stand (or sit) tall with abdominals pulled in.
Step both feet forward.

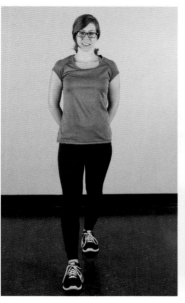
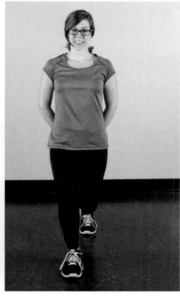

STEP 2
Step both feet back. Step forward and back for 1–2 minutes.

STEP 3
For added intensity, add a knee bend with the forward step.

JUMPING JACKS

Jumping jacks are a high-intensity, high-impact exercise. If neuropathy of the feet is present, modify exercise or do seated.

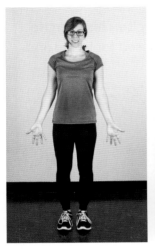 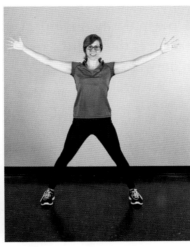

STEP 1

Stand (or sit) tall, abdominals pulled in. Jump feet out to either side while bringing arms up over head. Then return to start. Jump for 1–2 minutes.

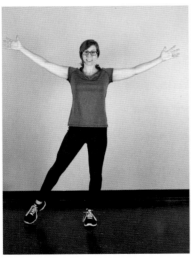 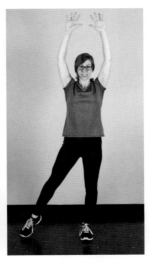

STEP 2

To modify, alternate side taps with feet while bringing arms up over head.

CHAPTER 5
Strength Exercises

BICEP CURLS

Bicep curls are a low-intensity, no-impact exercise. This exercise strengthens the front of the arm, the muscle used for lifting and rotating the arm outward.

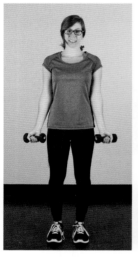 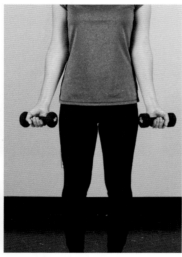

STEP 1
Stand (or sit) tall, feet at hip distance.

STEP 2
Put arms straight down by sides, palms facing up.

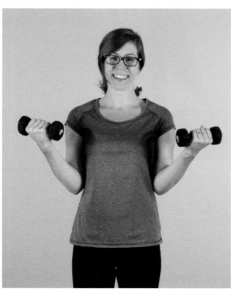

STEP 3
Keeping the elbows close to ribs, curl hands up towards shoulder.

STEP 4
The exercise can be done with one or both arms. Do 10–15 repetitions.

LATERAL RAISE

Lateral raises are a low-intensity, no-impact exercise. This exercise strengthens the shoulder muscles that are used for lifting and rotating the arms.

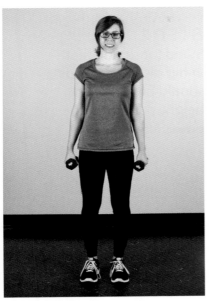

STEP 1

Stand (or sit) tall, feet at hip distance. Put arms straight down by sides, palms turned in toward body.

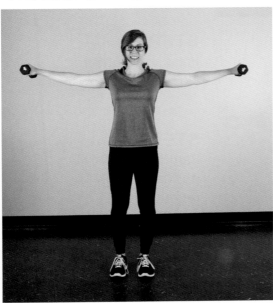

STEP 2

Lift one or both arms out to side, elbows slightly bent. Do not lift higher than the shoulder joint. Do 10–15 repetitions.

CHEST PRESS

This exercise is a low-intensity, no-impact exercise. The chest press will strengthen the chest muscles, which are important for pushing movements. This group of muscles also aids in maintaining good posture.

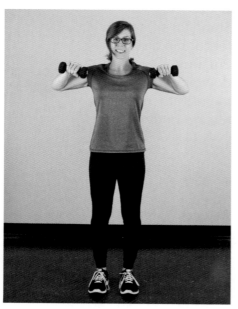

STEP 1
Stand (or sit) tall, feet at hip distance. Hands should be at chest height, palms facing down, elbows out.

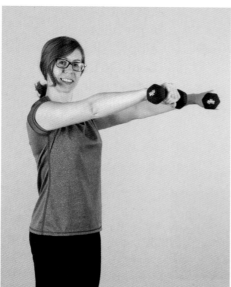

STEP 2
Press arms forward. Do not lock elbows.

STEP 3
Return to start position. Do 10–15 repetitions.

PRESS BACK

The press back is a low-intensity, no-impact exercise. This exercise strengthens the upper back muscles, which are important for pulling movements. This group of muscles also aids in maintaining good posture.

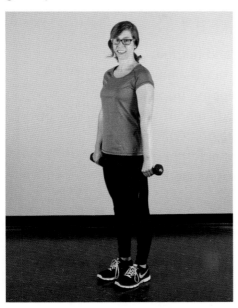

STEP 1

Stand (or sit) tall, feet at hip distance. Arms should be straight down by sides.

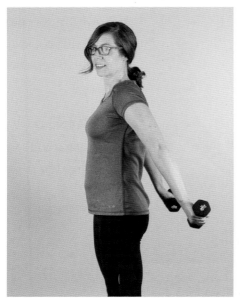

STEP 2

Face palms backward. Lift one or both arms back, squeezing shoulder blades. Keep shoulders relaxed. Do 10–15 repetitions.

SIDE LEG RAISE

This exercise is a low-intensity, no-impact exercise. Side raises strengthen the inner and outer thigh muscles, which are important for side to side movements. Be caution of this exercise if hip pain or injury is present.

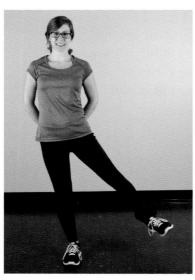

STEP 1

Stand tall, feet at hip distance. Keeping upper body tall, lift straight leg to the side. Keep foot relaxed.

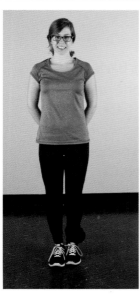 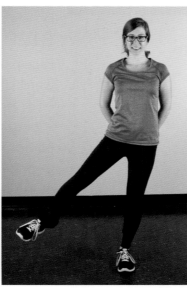

STEP 2

Return to start position. Do 10–15 repetitions.

STEP 3

Repeat with other leg.

LEG CURL

The leg curl exercise is a low-intensity, no-impact exercise. This exercise strengthens the muscles at the back of the thigh, which are important for bending the knee and walking. Be cautious if knee pain or injury is present. An ankle weight can be used.

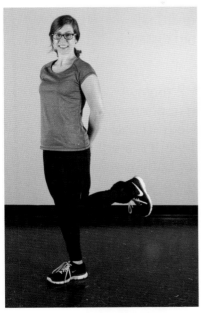

STEP 1

Stand tall, feet at hip distance. With left foot flexed, bend left knee, bringing foot backward.

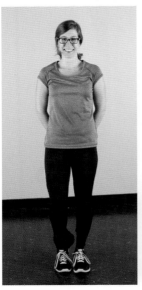
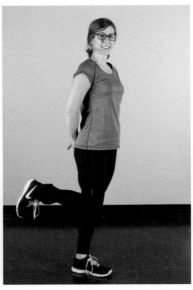

STEP 2

Keep knees close together. Lower to start position. Do 10–15 repetitions. Repeat with other leg.

HEEL RAISES

Heel raises are a low-intensity, low-impact exercise. This exercise strengthens the calf muscles. If neuropathy of the foot is present, do this exercise seated.

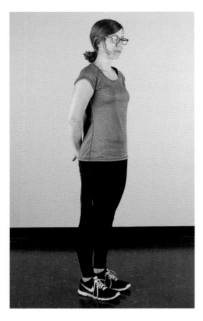

STEP 1
Stand (or sit) tall, feet at hip distance.

STEP 2 (below)
Keeping upper body tall and legs straight (knees bent, if seated), lift one or both heels off the ground. Do 10–15 repetitions.

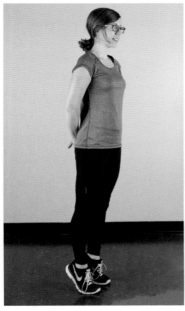

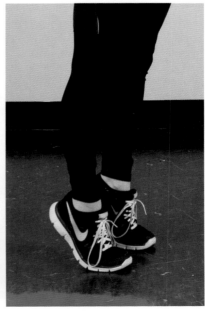

SQUATS

Squats are a moderate-intensity, no-impact exercise. Squats challenge all of the muscles of the upper leg, which are important for the fundamental movements of the lower body, such as walking, bending the knees, lifting the legs, and getting in and out of a chair. If hip or knee problems are present, do partial squats or avoid this exercise.

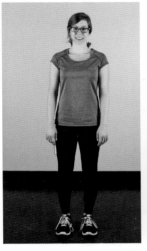 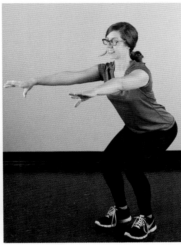

STEP 1
Stand with feet at hip distance. Pull in abdominals to protect lower back.

STEP 2
Bend knees and move hips back, as if sitting in a chair. Do not take knees farther forward than toes.

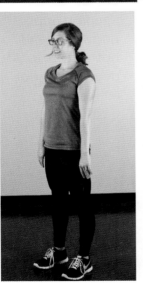

STEP 3
Press weight through heels to return to standing position. Do 10–15 repetitions.

LUNGES

Lunges are a moderate-intensity, no-impact exercise. This exercise strengthens the muscles of the thigh. If knee pain or injury is present, avoid this exercise.

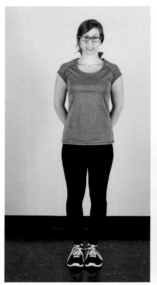 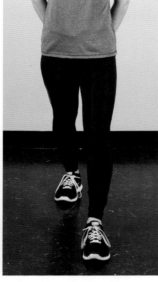

STEP 1
Stand tall with feet at hip distance. Step left foot forward into staggered stance.

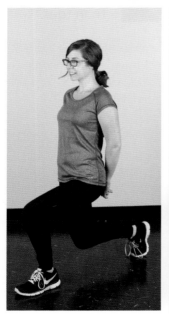 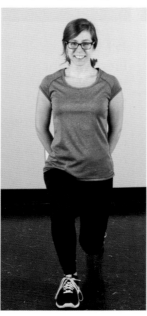

STEP 2
Keeping upper body tall, bend both knees to 90 degrees. Do not let knees go past the toes.

STEP 3
Return to standing position. Do 10–15 repetitions. Repeat with other leg.

LEG EXTENSIONS

Leg extensions on a stability ball are a double duty strength and balance exercise; they target the thigh muscles and the core. This low-intensity, no-impact exercise is safe for all fitness levels.

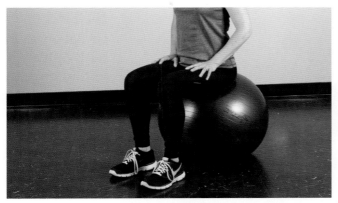

STEP 1

Sit on ball with feet flat on floor. Place hands on thighs. For more stability, place hands on either side of ball.

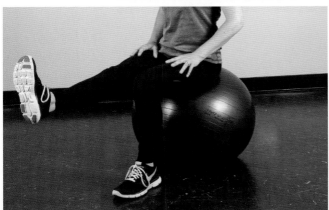

STEP 2

Sitting tall, lift right leg straight out, toes pointing to ceiling.

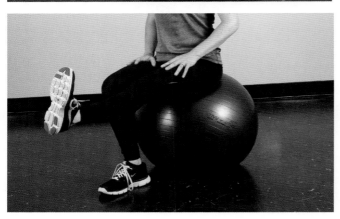

STEP 3

Lower to start position. Do 10–15 repetitions. Repeat with other leg.

HIP EXTENSIONS

Hip extensions target the hips and legs, both important muscles for walking. Adding the stability ball engages the core muscles and adds a balance challenge to the exercise. This is a no-impact, moderate-intensity exercise.

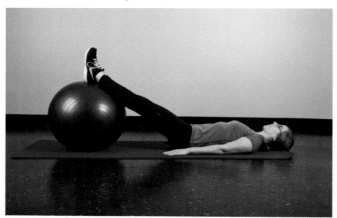

STEP 1

Lie flat on your back with ankles resting on a stability ball, legs straight.

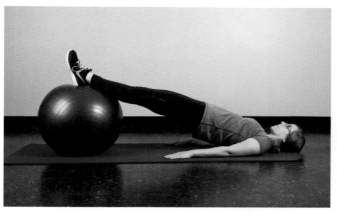

STEP 2

Keeping legs straight and abdominals contracted, lift hips towards ceiling. Keep neck and shoulders relaxed.

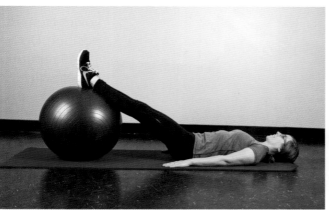

STEP 3

Pause for 1 count at the top of the lift. With firm abdominals, lower the hips back to the floor. Do 10–15 repetitions.

CHEST FLY

Chest fly exercises strengthen the muscles in the front of the chest. These muscles are key for good posture. This exercise is a moderate-intensity, no-impact exercise and is safe for all fitness levels. The addition of the ball incorporates core strength and balance.

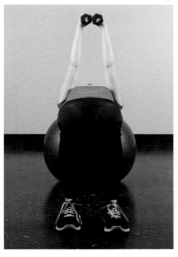

STEP 1
Sit on ball, feet at hip distance. Hold a 5–10 lb weight in each hand. Walk feet forward until upper back is resting on ball.

STEP 2
Straighten arms over head so hands are directly over the face, palms in. Arms should be nearly straight, keeping slight bend in elbows.

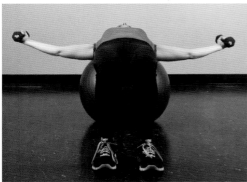

STEP 3
Lower arms out to sides, keeping elbows slightly bent.

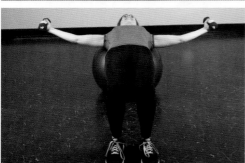

STEP 4
Return to start position. Do 10–15 repetitions.

TRICEP EXTENSION

This is a low-intensity, no-impact exercise. Tricep extensions work the back of the arms, strengthening the muscles in charge of pulling and pressing. The addition of the ball incorporates core strength and balance.

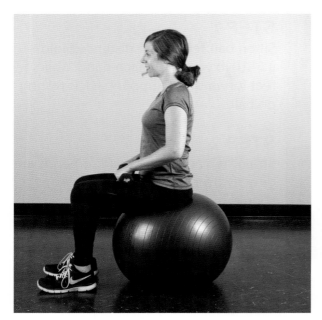

STEP 1

Sit on ball, feet at hip distance. Hold a 5–10 lb weight in each hand.

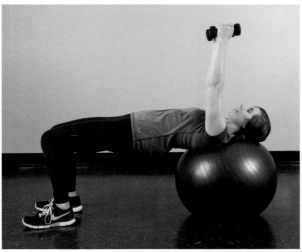

STEP 2

Walk feet forward until upper back is resting on ball. Keep hips lifted.

STEP 3

Straighten arms over head so hands are directly over the face, palms in. Arms should be straight.

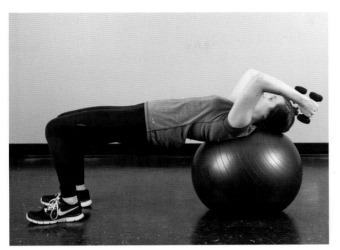

STEP 4

Bend elbows to 90 degrees, lowering hands behind head.

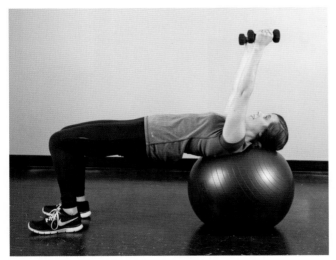

STEP 5

Press back to start position. Do 10–15 repetitions.

BRIDGE

This is a low-intensity, no-impact exercise targeting the lower body. The addition of the ball engages the core muscles and aids in balance training. Use caution if suffering from peripheral neuropathy.

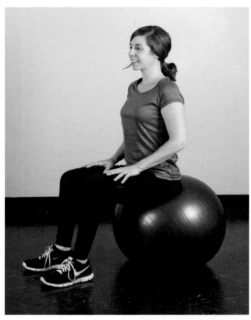

STEP 1
Sit on ball with feet flat on floor.

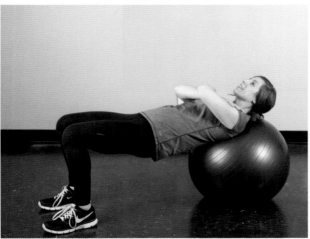

STEP 2
Walk the feet forward until upper body is resting on the ball, with knees bent at 90 degrees. Cross hands over chest.

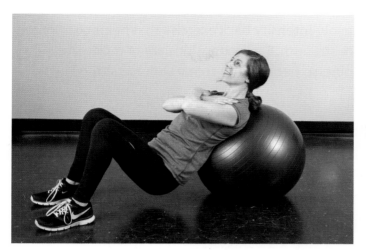

STEP 3
With tight abdominals, lower the hips until just above the floor.

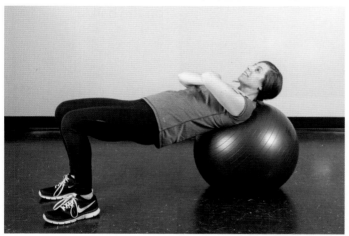

STEP 4
Keeping abdominals firm, press through the heels to lift the hips back to start position. Do 15 repetitions.

BACK EXTENSIONS

This exercise is a low-intensity back exercise that helps to improve posture and core strength. Back extensions are of moderate impact to the spine, so people with spinal stenosis should avoid this exercise.

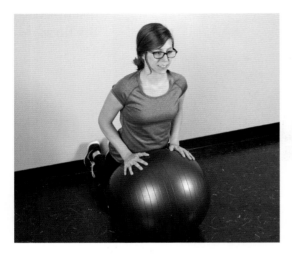

STEP 1

Bring the ball to an area with a wall nearby. Kneel in front of the ball. Lean forward, placing abdominals on the ball.

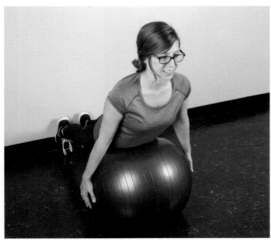

STEP 2

Straighten legs, securing feet against a wall.